Uterine Fibroids

A Step-by-Step Guide for Women to Managing Fibroids Through Diet and Other Natural Methods

copyright © 2024 Stephanie Hinderock

All rights reserved No part of this book may be reproduced, or stored in a retrieval system, or transmitted in any form or by any means, electronic, mechanical, photocopying, recording, or otherwise, without express written permission of the publisher.

Disclaimer

By reading this disclaimer, you are accepting the terms of the disclaimer in full. If you disagree with this disclaimer, please do not read the guide.

All of the content within this guide is provided for informational and educational purposes only, and should not be accepted as independent medical or other professional advice. The author is not a doctor, physician, nurse, mental health provider, or registered nutritionist/dietician. Therefore, using and reading this guide does not establish any form of a physician-patient relationship.

Always consult with a physician or another qualified health provider with any issues or questions you might have regarding any sort of medical condition. Do not ever disregard any qualified professional medical advice or delay seeking that advice because of anything you have read in this guide. The information in this guide is not intended to be any sort of medical advice and should not be used in lieu of any medical advice by a licensed and qualified medical professional.

The information in this guide has been compiled from a variety of known sources. However, the author cannot attest to or guarantee the accuracy of each source and thus should not be held liable for any errors or omissions.

You acknowledge that the publisher of this guide will not be held liable for any loss or damage of any kind incurred as a result of this guide or the reliance on any information provided within this guide. You acknowledge and agree that you assume all risk and responsibility for any action you undertake in response to the information in this guide.

Using this guide does not guarantee any particular result (e.g., weight loss or a cure). By reading this guide, you acknowledge that there are no guarantees to any specific outcome or results you can expect.

All product names, diet plans, or names used in this guide are for identification purposes only and are the property of their respective owners. The use of these names does not imply endorsement. All other trademarks cited herein are the property of their respective owners.

Where applicable, this guide is not intended to be a substitute for the original work of this diet plan and is, at most, a supplement to the original work for this diet plan and never a direct substitute. This guide is a personal expression of the facts of that diet plan.

Where applicable, persons shown in the cover images are stock photography models and the publisher has obtained the rights to use the images through license agreements with third-party stock image companies.

Table of Contents

Introduction — 7
Understanding Uterine Fibroids — 9
    Types of Uterine Fibroids — 9
    Evaluating Severity — 13
    Symptoms of Uterine Fibroids — 14
    When to See a Doctor — 20
    Causes and Risk Factors of Uterine Fibroids — 20
    Medical Treatments for Uterine Fibroids — 24
    Diagnosis of Uterine Fibroids — 28
    Natural Remedies for Uterine Fibroids — 35
Lifestyle Changes to Support Fibroid Management — 38
The Role of Diet in Managing Uterine Fibroids — 41
    Anti-inflammatory Foods — 41
    Limit High-Glycemic Foods — 43
    Reduce Red Meat Consumption — 47
    Increase Intake of Phytoestrogens — 50
    Foods to Eat for Managing Uterine Fibroids in Women — 54
    Foods to Avoid for Managing Uterine Fibroids in Women — 57
    Supplements — 60
Sample Recipes of Anti-inflammatory Food Diet to Manage Uterine Fibroids — 64
    Berry and Spinach Smoothie — 65
    Quinoa and Veggie Salad — 66
    Turmeric and Ginger Roasted Carrots — 67
    Salmon with Lemon and Dill — 68
    Sweet Potato and Black Bean Tacos — 69
    Kale and Chickpea Stir-Fry — 70
    Avocado and Tomato Salad — 71
    Lentil and Vegetable Soup — 72

Blueberry Chia Seed Pudding	73
Cucumber and Mint Infused Water	74
Grass-fed Beef Stew	75
Grilled Chicken Salad	76
Buckwheat Pancakes	77
Baked Salmon with Quinoa	79
Tofu Stir-Fry	80
Lentil Soup	82
Berry and Spinach Smoothie	83
Quinoa and Kale Salad	84
Baked Salmon with Asparagus	85
Sweet Potato and Black Bean Stew	86
Turmeric and Ginger Lentil Soup	87
7-Day Anti-Inflammatory Food Diet Sample Meal Plan	**89**
Conclusion	**92**
FAQs	**96**
References and Helpful Links	**99**

Introduction

Fibroids, also known as uterine leiomyomas, are noncancerous growths that develop within or on the uterus. These benign tumors are composed of muscle and fibrous tissue and can vary greatly in size. Some fibroids are so small they are undetectable by the human eye, while others can grow large enough to distort the shape and size of the uterus.

Uterine fibroids are a prevalent health condition affecting women of reproductive age. It is estimated that between 20% and 80% of women will develop fibroids by the time they reach the age of 50. While fibroids are most commonly diagnosed in women aged 30-40, they can occur at any age and across all racial and ethnic groups, though they are more common and tend to be more severe in African-American women.

Grasping the nuances of fibroid management is crucial due to the considerable effects these growths can have on a woman's well-being. Common symptoms such as excessive menstrual bleeding, pelvic discomfort, and fertility issues can deeply influence daily activities and overall health. Implementing suitable management techniques can help alleviate these symptoms, improve quality of life, and empower women to make informed choices regarding their healthcare options.

In this guide, we will talk about the following;

- Understanding Uterine Fibroids
- Lifestyle Changes to Support Fibroid Management
- The Role of Diet in Managing Uterine Fibroids
- Sample Recipes to Incorporate Anti-inflammatory Foods
- 7-Day Sample Meal Plan

By educating women on the many ways to manage fibroids, this guide aims to empower them to take control of their health and work in partnership with healthcare providers to find the best solutions for their individual needs.

Understanding Uterine Fibroids

Uterine fibroids, also known as leiomyomas or myomas, are benign growths that develop in the muscular wall of the uterus. They are made up of smooth muscle fibers and connective tissue and can vary in size from a pea to a melon. Sometimes they grow as individual tumors, while other times they form clusters or may even cover the entire surface of the uterus.

Fibroids can be classified into three types based on their location within the uterus: subserosal (outer wall), intramural (middle layer), or submucosal (inner layer). Some fibroids appear to hang like mushrooms inside or outside the uterus, while others grow into the uterine cavity. The size and location of fibroids can determine the types of symptoms experienced by a woman.

Types of Uterine Fibroids

Uterine Fibroids can develop in different locations within the uterus, leading to several types based on their position:

1. **Intramural Fibroids**

   Intramural fibroids are the most common type of uterine fibroids. These fibroids develop within the muscular wall, or myometrium, of the uterus. Due to their location within the muscle layer, they can cause the uterine walls to thicken and expand. This can lead to a variety of symptoms, including:

   - *Excessive Menstrual Bleeding*: Increased blood flow during periods due to the extra tissue in the uterine wall.
   - *Pelvic Discomfort and Pressure*: Discomfort caused by the enlargement of the uterine wall.
   - *Increased Urination Frequency*: Pressure on the bladder resulting from the enlarged uterine wall.
   - *Lumbar Pain*: Pain radiating to the lower back due to the pressure exerted by the fibroid.

2. **Submucosal Fibroids**

   Submucosal fibroids grow just under the lining, or endometrium, of the uterus. They can protrude into the uterine cavity, significantly impacting menstrual cycles and fertility. Common symptoms associated with submucosal fibroids include:

   - *Excessive or Extended Menstrual Bleeding*: Submucosal fibroids can increase the surface

area of the endometrium, leading to heavier and longer periods.
- *Anemia*: Chronic heavy bleeding can result in low levels of red blood cells, causing fatigue and weakness.
- *Infertility*: These fibroids can interfere with the implantation of an embryo or block the fallopian tubes.
- *Miscarriages*: Increased risk of miscarriage due to the distortion of the uterine cavity.

3. **Subserosal Fibroids**

Subserosal fibroids grow on the outer surface of the uterus, known as the serosa. They can become quite large and extend outward, affecting nearby organs. They often cause the following symptoms:

- *Pelvic Pain or Pressure*: Due to their size, subserosal fibroids can press against other organs, such as the bladder or rectum, causing discomfort.
- *Back and Leg Pain*: Large fibroids can exert pressure on nerves that extend to the lower back and legs.
- *Bloating and Abdominal Distension*: Visible swelling in the abdomen as the fibroid grows.
- *Constipation*: Pressure on the intestines can lead to difficulty in bowel movements.

4. Pedunculated Fibroids

Pedunculated fibroids are attached to the uterus by a stalk-like structure called a peduncle. These fibroids can form either inside (submucosal) or outside (subserosal) the uterus.

Depending on their location, they may cause unique symptoms:

- *Acute Pain*: If the peduncle twists, it can cut off the blood supply to the fibroid, causing severe pain.
- *Sudden Sharp Pain*: Due to the movement or growth of the fibroid itself.
- *Pressure Symptoms*: Similar to submucosal or subserosal fibroids, depending on their location.
- *Urinary or Bowel Issues*: Depending on the direction of their growth, they can press against the bladder or intestines, causing corresponding symptoms.

Understanding the type of fibroid and its specific symptoms is crucial for effective management and treatment. If you experience any of these symptoms, consult a healthcare provider for appropriate diagnosis and care.

Evaluating Severity

Assessing the severity of uterine fibroids is a crucial step in determining the most appropriate treatment plan. The evaluation process typically involves a combination of diagnostic imaging, symptom assessment, and consideration of the patient's overall health and reproductive goals. The following factors are taken into account:

Size of Fibroids

The size of fibroids can vary significantly, from as small as a pea to as large as a melon. The size is often measured in centimeters using imaging techniques such as ultrasound or MRI. Larger fibroids tend to cause more severe symptoms and may require more aggressive treatment.

- *Small Fibroids (<2 cm)*: Often asymptomatic and may not require immediate intervention.
- *Medium Fibroids (2-5 cm)*: Can cause moderate symptoms and may need medical management.
- *Large Fibroids (>5 cm)*: Typically associated with significant symptoms and may necessitate surgical treatment.

Number of Fibroids

The number of fibroids present in the uterus also plays a role in the severity of the condition. Multiple fibroids can compound symptoms and complicate treatment.

- *Single Fibroid*: Easier to manage and treat.
- *Multiple Fibroids*: May cause more severe symptoms and require comprehensive treatment plans.

Symptoms of Uterine Fibroids

The majority of women with uterine fibroids may not experience any symptoms, and the condition is often detected during a routine pelvic exam or imaging tests for another reason. However, some women may experience one or more of the following symptoms:

1. **Excessive Menstrual Bleeding**

    Excessive menstrual bleeding is the most common symptom associated with uterine fibroids. This condition, known medically as menorrhagia, can significantly impact a woman's quality of life. Symptoms include:

    - *Prolonged Periods*: Menstrual bleeding that lasts longer than seven days can be a sign of underlying health issues. This extended duration can cause significant discomfort and may require a medical evaluation to diagnose any potential conditions.
    - *Frequent Changing*: When blood flow is heavy enough to necessitate changing sanitary products every hour or even more frequently, it can disrupt daily activities and lead to anxiety

about leaks. This level of bleeding may indicate a need for further investigation to understand the cause.

- ***Clots***: The passage of large blood clots during menstruation can be alarming and often suggests a more serious condition. These clots, which can vary in size, may indicate a hormonal imbalance or other health issues that should be addressed by a healthcare professional.
- ***Anemia***: Chronic excessive bleeding can lead to anemia, a condition characterized by fatigue, weakness, and pale skin due to low red blood cell counts. This can significantly impact a person's quality of life, making it essential to monitor symptoms and seek treatment to restore proper iron levels and overall health.

2. Pelvic Pressure or Pain

Fibroids can cause a sensation of fullness or pressure in the pelvic area, along with varying degrees of pain. This discomfort arises from the fibroids pressing against nearby organs and tissues, leading to:

- ***Lower Abdominal Fullness***: This sensation often manifests as a feeling of heaviness or pressure in the lower abdomen, which can be quite similar to bloating. It may result from the presence of fibroids that can distort the normal

abdominal contour, leading to discomfort and an overall sensation of fullness.
- ***Dull or Sharp Pain***: Individuals may experience consistent dull aches that can become quite bothersome, or they may encounter intermittent sharp pains that vary based on the size and location of the fibroids. These pains can impact daily activities and can vary in intensity, making it crucial to monitor their occurrence.
- ***Pain During Activities***: Many people report increased discomfort during physical activities, such as exercise or even simple tasks like walking or lifting. Prolonged standing can also exacerbate this discomfort, making it important to listen to your body and adjust activities accordingly when fibroids are present.

3. **Frequent Urination**

Fibroids located near the bladder can exert pressure on this organ, leading to urinary symptoms such as:

- ***Increased Urgency***: A sudden and compelling need to urinate that can strike unexpectedly, often leading to discomfort or anxiety if a restroom isn't nearby. This sensation can be intense and may feel overwhelming, making it difficult to focus on other activities.

- *Frequent Urination*: The need to urinate more often than usual can be disruptive to daily life, as it may interrupt work, social engagements, and even restful sleep. This increased frequency can leave individuals feeling frustrated and constantly on the lookout for the nearest bathroom.
- *Small Volumes*: Many people experience frequent urges to urinate, but when they actually go, they may only pass small amounts of urine each time. This phenomenon can lead to a feeling of incomplete relief and can exacerbate the urgency, creating a cycle of discomfort and frequent visits to the restroom.

4. Difficulty Emptying Your Bladder

Large fibroids can obstruct the normal flow of urine, causing difficulties in properly emptying the bladder:

- *Incomplete Emptying*: Feeling that the bladder isn't fully emptied after urination.
- *Urinary Hesitancy*: Difficulty starting the flow of urine or prolonged duration to initiate urination.
- *Weak Stream*: A decrease in the strength of the urinary stream.

5. **Constipation**

   Fibroids that grow outward and press against the bowel can interfere with normal digestive processes, leading to:

   - *Bowel Compression*: Pressure on the intestines, causing them to narrow and making it harder for stools to pass.
   - *Difficulty Passing Stools*: Straining during bowel movements and experiencing hard or lumpy stools.
   - *Bloating*: Feeling of fullness and bloating due to delayed or incomplete bowel movements.

6. **Backache**

   Fibroids growing on the outer wall of the uterus can exert pressure on nerves that extend to the back, leading to:

   - *Lower Back Pain*: Persistent or intermittent pain in the lower back region.
   - *Radiating Pain*: Pain that may radiate to the legs or hips, mimicking sciatica symptoms.
   - *Aggravated by Movement*: Pain that worsens with prolonged standing, walking, or certain physical activities.

7. Pain During Sex

Submucosal fibroids, which protrude into the uterine cavity, can cause discomfort or pain during sexual intercourse:

- ***Deep Dyspareunia***: This condition is characterized by pain experienced during deep penetration, often described as a deep, aching sensation that can be distressing and interfere with sexual enjoyment. It may stem from various underlying issues, including pelvic floor dysfunction or endometriosis, and requires careful evaluation and management.
- ***Positional Pain***: Some individuals experience variation in pain intensity depending on the sexual positions used. Certain positions may exacerbate discomfort, while others might provide relief. Understanding which positions work best can enhance sexual experiences and foster better communication between partners.
- ***Emotional Impact***: Chronic pain during sex can take a significant toll on mental health, leading to anxiety, stress, and reduced sexual desire over time. This emotional burden can create a cycle of distress that affects relationships and overall well-being, making it crucial to address

both the physical and emotional aspects of sexual health.

Understanding these symptoms can help in recognizing the presence of fibroids and seeking timely medical attention. If you experience any of these symptoms, consult a healthcare provider for appropriate diagnosis and treatment options.

When to See a Doctor

It is essential to consult a healthcare provider if you experience symptoms that interfere with your daily life or well-being. Seek medical advice if you notice:

- Excessive Menstrual Bleeding
- Severe pelvic pain
- Difficulty emptying the bladder
- Symptoms of anemia, such as fatigue and shortness of breath
- Any changes in your menstrual cycle or unusual bleeding patterns

Early diagnosis and intervention can help manage symptoms effectively and prevent complications.

Causes and Risk Factors of Uterine Fibroids

The exact cause of uterine fibroids remains unknown. However, several factors have been identified that may increase a woman's risk of developing these benign tumors.

Understanding these factors is crucial for early detection and management.

1. **Age**

   Fibroids are most common in women aged 30 to 40 years old. As women approach their reproductive peak and mid-life, their risk of developing fibroids increases. This age group is particularly susceptible due to:

   - *Hormonal Fluctuations*: As women age, especially during their reproductive years, they experience significant hormonal changes that can influence the growth of fibroids.
   - *Menstrual Cycles*: The cumulative effect of multiple menstrual cycles over the years may contribute to the development of fibroids.

2. **Family History**

   A family history of uterine fibroids significantly increases the likelihood of developing them. If a first-degree relative (mother or sister) has fibroids, your chances are higher due to:

   - *Genetic Predisposition*: Certain genes may predispose women to develop fibroids, inherited from their parents.
   - *Shared Environmental Factors*: Lifestyle and environmental factors shared within families,

such as diet and stress levels, can also play a role.

3. **Ethnicity**

African American women have a higher risk of fibroids compared to women of other ethnicities. This increased risk can be attributed to:

- *Genetic Factors*: Genetic variations that are more prevalent in African American women may contribute to the development and growth of fibroids.
- *Earlier Onset*: African American women tend to develop fibroids at a younger age and are more likely to experience severe symptoms.
- *Higher Incidence*: Studies show that African American women are two to three times more likely to develop fibroids than women of other races.

4. **Obesity**

Women who are overweight or obese are more likely to develop fibroids. The connection between obesity and fibroids is linked to:

- *Excess Estrogen*: Fat cells produce estrogen, and higher levels of body fat can lead to increased estrogen production, which may stimulate fibroid growth.

- ***Insulin Resistance***: Obesity is often associated with insulin resistance, which can influence hormone levels and contribute to fibroid development.
- ***Inflammation***: Chronic low-grade inflammation common in obesity may promote the growth of fibroids.

5. Hormonal Imbalances

Estrogen and progesterone are hormones that regulate the menstrual cycle and play a role in the development of fibroids. An imbalance in these hormones can contribute to fibroid growth through several mechanisms:

- ***Estrogen Dominance***: Elevated levels of estrogen, without the counterbalancing effect of progesterone, can stimulate the growth of fibroid tissue.
- ***Progesterone Sensitivity***: Fibroids have been found to contain more receptors for estrogen and progesterone than normal uterine muscle cells, making them more sensitive to these hormones.
- ***Menstrual Cycle Variations***: Irregularities in the menstrual cycle, influenced by hormonal imbalances, can create an environment conducive to fibroid growth.

Understanding these risk factors can help women take proactive steps in monitoring their health and seeking medical advice when necessary. Early detection and intervention can significantly improve the management of uterine fibroids and enhance overall well-being.

Medical Treatments for Uterine Fibroids

There are various medical treatments available for uterine fibroids, depending on the severity of symptoms and individual needs. Some common treatment options include:

1. **Medications**

    Medications can be an effective way to manage the symptoms of uterine fibroids. These may include:

    - *Hormonal Birth Control Pills*: These pills can help regulate menstrual cycles, reduce excessive bleeding, and alleviate pain. Options include combined oral contraceptives containing both estrogen and progestin or progestin-only pills.
    - *Progestin-Releasing Intrauterine Device (IUD)*: This device releases a small amount of progestin into the uterus, which can thin the uterine lining and reduce menstrual bleeding.
    - *Other Hormonal Medications*: Medications such as danazol, which suppresses the production of estrogen and progesterone, can reduce the size of fibroids and lessen bleeding.

2. **Nonsteroidal Anti-Inflammatory Drugs (NSAIDs)**

   NSAIDs are commonly used to relieve pain and discomfort caused by fibroids. These over-the-counter or prescription medications include:

   - *Ibuprofen and Naproxen*: These drugs can help alleviate menstrual cramps and reduce inflammation.
   - *Effectiveness*: While NSAIDs do not shrink fibroids, they can significantly improve quality of life by managing pain and reducing the need for stronger pain medications.
   - *Usage*: Typically taken during menstruation or as needed for pain relief.

3. **Gonadotropin-Releasing Hormone (GnRH) Agonists**

   GnRH agonists are a class of drugs that temporarily shrink fibroids by reducing estrogen levels in the body. They work by:

   - ***Suppressing Estrogen Production***: GnRH agonists lower estrogen and progesterone levels, mimicking a menopausal state, which leads to the temporary shrinkage of fibroids.
   - ***Short-Term Use***: These medications are usually prescribed for a short duration (typically 3-6 months) due to potential side effects like bone

loss and menopausal symptoms (hot flashes, night sweats).
- ***Pre-Surgical Treatment***: Often used before surgery to reduce the size of fibroids, making them easier to remove and minimizing surgical risks.

4. **Uterine Artery Embolization (UAE)**

Uterine artery embolization is a minimally invasive procedure that targets fibroids by cutting off their blood supply. Key aspects include:

- ***Procedure***: A radiologist inserts a catheter into the arteries supplying blood to the uterus and injects small particles to block these vessels, causing the fibroids to shrink and die.
- ***Recovery***: Patients typically require a short hospital stay and a few days of rest at home.
- ***Effectiveness***: UAE can reduce fibroid symptoms in many women without the need for major surgery, though it might not be suitable for those planning future pregnancies.

5. **Myomectomy**

Myomectomy is a surgical procedure designed to remove fibroids while preserving the uterus. It is often recommended for women who wish to become pregnant in the future. Types of myomectomy include:

- *Abdominal Myomectomy*: An open surgery where an incision is made in the lower abdomen to remove fibroids.
- *Laparoscopic Myomectomy*: A minimally invasive surgery using small incisions and a camera to guide the removal of fibroids.
- *Hysteroscopic Myomectomy*: A procedure performed through the vagina and cervix to remove fibroids from inside the uterine cavity.
- *Recovery*: Recovery time varies depending on the type of myomectomy, ranging from a few days to several weeks.

6. **Hysterectomy**

In severe cases where other treatments have been ineffective, a hysterectomy may be recommended. This involves the removal of the uterus and is considered a last resort. Key points include:

Types of Hysterectomy:

- *Total Hysterectomy*: Removal of the entire uterus, including the cervix.
- *Subtotal Hysterectomy*: Removal of the upper part of the uterus, leaving the cervix intact.
- *Radical Hysterectomy*: Removal of the uterus, cervix, part of the vagina, and surrounding tissues, usually for cancer treatment.

Consequences: A hysterectomy eliminates the possibility of future pregnancy and induces menopause if the ovaries are removed.

Recovery: Major surgery with a recovery period of several weeks to months, depending on the extent of the procedure.

Each of these treatments has its own benefits and potential risks. Women experiencing symptoms of uterine fibroids should consult their healthcare provider to determine the most appropriate treatment plan based on their individual needs and circumstances.

It is important to consult with a healthcare provider before deciding on a treatment plan for uterine fibroids. They can help determine the best course of action based on individual needs and preferences.

Diagnosis of Uterine Fibroids

Uterine fibroids, also known as leiomyomas or myomas, are non-cancerous growths that develop in or on the uterus. The diagnosis process typically involves a range of medical evaluations to confirm the presence of fibroids and assess their size, number, and location. Here is an expanded overview of the methods used to diagnose uterine fibroids:

1. **Pelvic Examination**

    A pelvic examination is often the first step in diagnosing uterine fibroids. During this thorough and careful exam, the healthcare provider will manually assess the size and shape of the uterus by palpating (feeling) the abdomen and internal organs. This process involves the provider using their hands to gently press on the abdomen to identify any abnormalities.

If an enlarged or irregularly shaped uterus is detected, it may raise suspicion of the presence of fibroids. This finding typically prompts further diagnostic tests, such as ultrasound imaging or MRI, to confirm the diagnosis and assess the size and location of the fibroids. By conducting a pelvic examination, healthcare providers can gather crucial information to guide appropriate treatment options and ensure the best care for the patient.

2. **Imaging Tests**

Imaging tests are essential diagnostic tools that provide detailed pictures of the inside of the body, allowing healthcare professionals to confirm diagnoses and gather vital information about the characteristics of fibroids. These tests not only help visualize the fibroids but also provide insights into their size, location, and potential impact on surrounding tissues. Common imaging techniques used in this context include:

Ultrasound (Sonography)

- ***Transabdominal Ultrasound***: In this non-invasive procedure, a device called a transducer is gently moved over the abdomen. It emits sound waves that bounce off internal structures, creating real-time images of the uterus and surrounding organs. This method is particularly useful for assessing the overall reproductive system and identifying larger fibroids.
- ***Transvaginal Ultrasound***: For a more detailed view, a transducer is carefully inserted into the vagina. This method allows for closer proximity to the uterus, providing clearer and more accurate images of the uterine structure and any fibroids present. Transvaginal ultrasound is often preferred when detailed assessment is required, especially for smaller fibroids or when evaluating the uterine lining.

These imaging techniques play a crucial role in the diagnosis and management of fibroids, guiding treatment decisions and helping to ensure the best possible outcomes for patients.

Ultrasound is often the first imaging test used due to its accessibility, safety, and effectiveness in visualizing fibroids.

3. **Magnetic Resonance Imaging (MRI)**

   Magnetic Resonance Imaging (MRI) is a non-invasive imaging technique that employs strong magnetic fields and radio waves to generate highly detailed images of the uterus and surrounding tissues. This advanced imaging modality is particularly beneficial for accurately mapping the size, number, and precise location of fibroids, which are non-cancerous growths that can develop in the uterus.

   MRI is especially valuable in cases where ultrasound results are inconclusive or when a more comprehensive imaging approach is required for effective treatment planning. By providing a clearer visualization of the fibroids, MRI helps healthcare professionals tailor treatment strategies, ensuring better outcomes for patients. Additionally, MRI does not involve ionizing radiation, making it a safe option for patients needing multiple imaging assessments.

4. **Computed Tomography (CT) Scan**

   CT scans, or computed tomography scans, utilize X-rays to generate detailed cross-sectional images of the body's internal structures. Although they are less frequently employed for diagnosing fibroids when compared to ultrasound and MRI, CT scans can still play a significant role in specific clinical scenarios.

For instance, they may be particularly useful in complex cases where additional anatomical detail is necessary, such as assessing the size and location of fibroids in relation to surrounding organs, or when there are concerns about possible complications. This added information can be crucial for healthcare providers in developing a comprehensive treatment plan tailored to the patient's unique needs.

5. **Other Diagnostic Procedures**

In some cases, additional procedures may be performed to gather more information or rule out other conditions that could be affecting a patient's reproductive health. These procedures can provide critical insights and help inform treatment decisions:

- *Hysterosonography (Saline Infusion Sonography)*

    This procedure involves injecting sterile saline into the uterine cavity during an ultrasound examination. By doing this, healthcare providers can obtain a clearer and more detailed view of the uterine lining and any fibroids present. The saline acts as a contrast agent, enhancing the visibility of the uterus and helping to identify irregularities that might not be seen in a standard ultrasound.

- **Hysteroscopy**

  During a hysteroscopy, a thin, flexible tube equipped with a camera, known as a hysteroscope, is carefully inserted through the vagina and cervix into the uterus. This minimally invasive procedure allows for direct visualization of the uterine cavity, providing doctors the opportunity to closely inspect the interior for any abnormalities. Hysteroscopy is particularly useful for identifying submucosal fibroids, which are those fibroids growing just beneath the inner lining of the uterus, as well as other conditions such as polyps or uterine adhesions that might be causing symptoms.

- **Endometrial Biopsy**

  An endometrial biopsy involves taking a small sample of the uterine lining, or endometrium, for laboratory analysis. This procedure is crucial for diagnosing various conditions, as it allows pathologists to examine the tissue under a microscope. Endometrial biopsies are often performed to rule out serious issues such as endometrial hyperplasia (an abnormal thickening of the uterine lining) or cancer, especially in patients presenting with abnormal uterine bleeding. The results from the biopsy can guide further management and treatment plans tailored to the individual's specific health needs.

6. **Lab Tests**

   Blood tests may sometimes be ordered to check for anemia, which can be a possible consequence of excessive menstrual bleeding associated with uterine fibroids. Anemia occurs when the body lacks enough red blood cells to carry adequate oxygen to tissues, leading to fatigue and weakness. These blood tests can also help identify other underlying health issues that may contribute to the symptoms experienced by the patient.

The diagnosis of uterine fibroids typically involves a comprehensive approach, combining clinical examinations, such as pelvic exams, with imaging tests like ultrasounds or MRIs to visualize the fibroids and assess their size and location. In some cases, healthcare providers may recommend invasive procedures, such as hysteroscopy or laparoscopy, to obtain more detailed information about the fibroids and the overall condition of the uterus.

Early and accurate diagnosis is essential, as it allows for timely intervention and is crucial for determining the most effective course of treatment, whether that involves medication, lifestyle changes, or surgical options, ultimately aiding in the effective management of symptoms and improving the patient's quality of life.

Natural Remedies for Uterine Fibroids

Here are some natural remedies that may help manage uterine fibroids, focusing solely on dietary and herbal approaches:

1. ***Green Tea***: Green tea is packed with beneficial compounds, particularly epigallocatechin gallate (EGCG), which is known for its impressive anti-inflammatory and antiproliferative effects. Research suggests that these properties may help to reduce both the size and number of uterine fibroids, making green tea a valuable addition to a health-conscious diet for those managing fibroid-related issues.
2. ***Turmeric***: Turmeric contains curcumin, a powerful compound celebrated for its strong anti-inflammatory properties. By combating inflammation, curcumin can inhibit the growth of fibroid cells, potentially slowing their development and providing relief from associated pain. Incorporating turmeric into meals or taking it as a supplement might offer significant benefits for individuals dealing with fibroids.
3. ***Milk Thistle***: Milk thistle is renowned for its liver detoxifying capabilities, which are crucial for maintaining hormone balance in the body. By

supporting liver function and helping to regulate estrogen levels, milk thistle can play a beneficial role in managing fibroids and their symptoms. Many people choose to take milk thistle as a supplement to promote overall liver health.

4. ***Dandelion Root***: Dandelion root is a natural remedy that aids in liver detoxification, promoting the efficient elimination of toxins from the body. It also helps to balance hormone levels by enhancing the body's ability to remove excess estrogen, which can contribute to fibroid growth. Consuming dandelion root tea or supplements may provide a holistic approach to hormone regulation.

5. ***Chasteberry (Vitex)***: Chasteberry is a herb commonly used in traditional medicine to help balance hormones. It is particularly effective for women experiencing symptoms related to uterine fibroids, as it influences the pituitary gland to regulate hormone production. This hormonal balance can alleviate discomfort and may even reduce the size of fibroids over time.

6. ***Ginger***: Known for its culinary versatility, ginger also boasts remarkable anti-inflammatory and antioxidant properties. Regular consumption of ginger can help alleviate pain and reduce inflammation associated with fibroids. Whether incorporated into meals, brewed as a tea, or taken in supplement form, ginger can be a soothing addition to a fibroid management plan.

7. ***Garlic***: Garlic is not only a flavorful ingredient but also a powerhouse of antioxidants with notable anti-inflammatory effects. Its ability to combat inflammation can be particularly helpful for those managing fibroid symptoms. Incorporating fresh garlic into your diet or taking garlic supplements may help inhibit the growth of fibroids while promoting overall health.

By incorporating these natural remedies into your routine, you can support the management of uterine fibroids in a holistic way.

Lifestyle Changes to Support Fibroid Management

1. *Maintain a Healthy Weight*: Excess body weight can lead to higher estrogen levels, which may contribute to the growth of uterine fibroids. Maintaining a balanced diet rich in fruits, vegetables, whole grains, and lean proteins is crucial. Pair this with regular physical activity, such as walking, running, or group sports, to achieve and sustain a healthy weight. It's important to monitor portion sizes and avoid highly processed foods that can lead to weight gain.

2. *Regular Exercise*: Engaging in regular physical activity not only helps regulate hormones but also reduces inflammation, which can be beneficial for those with fibroids. Aim for at least 30 minutes of moderate exercise, such as brisk walking, swimming, cycling, or group fitness classes, on most days of the week to improve overall health and well-being. Incorporating strength training exercises a few times a

week can further enhance your fitness level and hormone regulation.

3. **Stress Management**: Chronic stress can significantly disrupt hormonal balance, potentially worsening fibroid symptoms. It's essential to incorporate stress-relieving activities into your daily routine. Consider practices such as:

4. **Yoga and Meditation**: These practices promote relaxation, enhance mental well-being, and help in lowering stress levels. Regular classes, whether in-person or online, can provide structure and motivation.

5. **Mindfulness Techniques**: Techniques like deep breathing exercises, progressive muscle relaxation, and mindfulness meditation can effectively help manage stress and promote a sense of calm.

6. **Avoid Environmental Toxins**: Certain chemicals found in everyday items like plastics, pesticides, and personal care products can mimic estrogen in the body, potentially exacerbating the growth of fibroids. To reduce exposure, consider the following strategies:

7. **Choosing Natural Products**: Opt for organic produce whenever possible, as they are less likely to contain harmful pesticides. Additionally, select natural

skincare and cleaning products that are free from synthetic chemicals.

8. ***Using Glass or Stainless Steel Containers***: Instead of plastic for food and drink storage, using glass or stainless steel containers can minimize your exposure to harmful chemicals that leach from plastic. This simple switch can make a significant difference in reducing your overall toxin load.

Managing uterine fibroids through diet and lifestyle involves making informed and proactive choices. By incorporating anti-inflammatory foods, limiting high-glycemic and red meat consumption, increasing phytoestrogen intake, and adopting healthy lifestyle habits, you can create a supportive environment for reducing fibroid symptoms and enhancing overall well-being. Remember, while these strategies can be beneficial, it's essential to consult with your healthcare provider for personalized advice and treatment plans tailored to your specific needs.

The Role of Diet in Managing Uterine Fibroids

Incorporating certain dietary changes can play a significant role in managing uterine fibroids. Here are some key points to consider:

Anti-inflammatory Foods

Inflammation is linked to the development and growth of fibroids. Incorporating anti-inflammatory foods into your diet can help reduce inflammation and potentially slow the progression of fibroids. Here's a detailed look at key anti-inflammatory foods:

Fruits and Vegetables

Fruits and vegetables are powerhouses of antioxidants, vitamins, and minerals that combat inflammation and promote overall health. Some particularly beneficial choices include:

- *Leafy Greens*: Spinach, kale, and Swiss chard are loaded with vitamins A, C, and K, which have potent anti-inflammatory properties.
- *Berries*: Blueberries, strawberries, and raspberries are rich in flavonoids and antioxidants like anthocyanins, which help neutralize harmful free radicals and reduce inflammation.
- *Citrus Fruits*: Oranges, grapefruits, and lemons provide a high dose of vitamin C, an antioxidant that plays a critical role in reducing inflammation.
- *Cruciferous Vegetables*: Broccoli, cauliflower, Brussels sprouts, and cabbage contain sulforaphane, a compound that has been shown to have anti-inflammatory and cancer-fighting properties.

Healthy Fats

Healthy fats are essential for reducing inflammation in the body. They support cellular function, hormone production, and overall wellness. Key sources include:

- *Avocados*: Packed with monounsaturated fats, avocados also contain fiber, potassium, and magnesium, which help reduce blood pressure and inflammation.
- *Olive Oil*: Extra virgin olive oil is rich in oleic acid and polyphenols, compounds known for their powerful anti-inflammatory effects.

- ***Fatty Fish***: Salmon, mackerel, sardines, and trout are excellent sources of omega-3 fatty acids, which have been extensively studied for their ability to lower inflammation by decreasing the production of inflammatory molecules called cytokines.

Whole Grains

Whole grains are high in fiber and nutrients that help maintain hormonal balance and support digestive health. They can play a crucial role in managing fibroid symptoms by regulating blood sugar levels and promoting a healthy gut microbiome. Some nutrient-dense whole grains include:

- ***Brown Rice***: A great source of magnesium, selenium, and B vitamins, brown rice helps support metabolic functions and reduce systemic inflammation.
- ***Quinoa***: This gluten-free grain is packed with protein, fiber, and antioxidants like quercetin and kaempferol, which have notable anti-inflammatory properties.
- ***Oats***: Rich in beta-glucan, a type of soluble fiber, oats help lower cholesterol levels and improve immune response, contributing to reduced inflammation.

Limit High-Glycemic Foods

High-glycemic foods can spike insulin levels, potentially contributing to hormonal imbalances and the growth of fibroids. By limiting these foods, you can help manage your blood sugar levels, support hormone regulation, and reduce the risk of fibroid development.

Here's a deeper look into what to avoid and healthier alternatives:

Refined Sugars

Refined sugars are quickly absorbed into the bloodstream, leading to rapid spikes in blood sugar and insulin levels. These fluctuations can contribute to hormonal imbalances that may exacerbate fibroid growth. Common sources of refined sugars include:

- *Candies*: Often loaded with high amounts of sugar and lacking any nutritional value, candies can cause significant insulin spikes.
- *Pastries*: Baked goods like cakes, cookies, and donuts are not only high in sugar but also in unhealthy fats, which can further promote inflammation.
- *Sugary Drinks*: Beverages such as sodas, sweetened iced teas, energy drinks, and fruit juices contain large quantities of added sugars. For instance, just one 12-ounce can of soda can contain up to 10 teaspoons of sugar.

Healthier Alternatives:

- *Natural Sweeteners*: Opt for natural sweeteners like honey, maple syrup, or stevia in moderation.

- ***Whole Fruits***: Satisfy your sweet tooth with whole fruits, which contain natural sugars along with fiber, vitamins, and minerals.

Processed Foods

Processed foods often have a high glycemic index due to the refining process, which strips away essential nutrients and fiber. This can lead to rapid increases in blood sugar levels and contribute to hormonal disruptions. Common processed foods to limit include:

- ***White Bread***: Made from refined flour, white bread has a high glycemic index and lacks the fiber and nutrients found in whole grains.
- ***Pasta***: Regular pasta made from refined wheat flour can cause blood sugar spikes. Whole grain or alternative pasta (like those made from chickpeas or lentils) are better options.
- ***Snack Foods***: Items like chips, crackers, and certain breakfast cereals are often high in refined sugars, unhealthy fats, and additives. They offer little nutritional value and can disrupt blood sugar balance.

Healthier Alternatives:

- ***Whole Grain Products***: Choose whole grain versions of bread, pasta, and rice, which contain more fiber and nutrients that help regulate blood sugar levels.

- *Homemade Snacks*: Prepare snacks at home using whole ingredients, such as raw nuts, seeds, and homemade granola bars without added sugars.

Practical Tips for Reducing High-Glycemic Foods

- *Read Labels Carefully*: Check the nutrition labels on packaged foods to identify hidden sugars and refined ingredients. Look for terms like sucrose, glucose, high-fructose corn syrup, and maltose.
- *Cook at Home*: Preparing meals at home allows you to control the ingredients and avoid high-glycemic foods. Focus on cooking with whole, unprocessed ingredients.
- *Plan Balanced Meals*: Include a mix of protein, healthy fats, and fiber-rich carbohydrates in your meals to help stabilize blood sugar levels and keep you feeling full longer.
- *Stay Hydrated*: Sometimes thirst is mistaken for hunger, leading to unhealthy snacking. Drink plenty of water throughout the day to stay hydrated and support metabolic processes.

By limiting high-glycemic foods, you can better manage insulin levels and maintain hormonal balance, which is crucial for controlling the growth and symptoms of uterine fibroids. Incorporating natural sweeteners, whole grains, and nutrient-dense snacks into your diet can further support your overall health and well-being.

Reduce Red Meat Consumption

Studies suggest that high consumption of red meat may be linked to an increased risk of developing fibroids. While the exact mechanisms are still being researched, red meat often contains added hormones and is associated with inflammation, both of which can contribute to fibroid growth. By reducing red meat intake and opting for lean protein sources, you can support better hormonal balance and overall health.

Here's a deeper dive into why and how to make these dietary changes:

The Link Between Red Meat and Fibroids

Red meat, particularly when consumed in large quantities, has several characteristics that may contribute to fibroid development:

- *Hormonal Content*: Some red meats contain added hormones, or they can influence the body's hormone levels, potentially leading to imbalances that promote fibroid growth.
- *Inflammatory Properties*: Red meat is high in saturated fats, which can increase inflammation in the body. Chronic inflammation is a known risk factor for the development and growth of fibroids.

- ***Iron Overload***: Excessive consumption of red meat can lead to elevated iron levels, which might contribute to oxidative stress and inflammation.

Healthier Protein Alternatives

Opting for lean, plant-based, or other healthier protein sources can help mitigate the risks associated with red meat. These options are typically lower in saturated fats and free from added hormones, promoting a more balanced diet conducive to fibroid management.

- ***Poultry***: Chicken and turkey are excellent sources of lean protein. They provide essential amino acids without the high levels of saturated fats found in red meat. Opt for skinless, white meat portions like chicken breast, and prepare them using healthy cooking methods such as grilling, baking, or steaming.
- ***Fish***: Fatty fish like salmon, mackerel, and sardines are rich in omega-3 fatty acids, which have anti-inflammatory properties that can help reduce inflammation and support heart health. Other types of fish, such as cod and tilapia, also offer lean protein with minimal fat.
- ***Tofu***: Made from soybeans, tofu is a versatile and protein-rich option for those looking to reduce animal protein intake. It is low in saturated fats and contains phytoestrogens, which may help balance hormone

levels. Use tofu in stir-fries, soups, or as a meat substitute in various dishes.
- **_Legumes_**: Beans, lentils, chickpeas, and peas are excellent sources of plant-based protein and fiber. They help maintain stable blood sugar levels and provide important nutrients like iron, magnesium, and folate. Incorporate legumes into salads, soups, stews, and grain bowls.

Practical Tips for Reducing Red Meat Intake

- **_Gradual Reduction_**: If you're accustomed to eating red meat frequently, start by reducing the number of times you consume it each week. Aim to replace red meat with lean proteins or plant-based alternatives progressively.
- **_Meatless Meals_**: Designate certain days of the week as "meatless" to encourage the exploration of vegetarian or vegan meals. This can help diversify your diet and introduce you to new, nutrient-rich foods.
- **_Portion Control_**: When you do consume red meat, keep portions small and choose the leanest cuts available. Trim any visible fat before cooking.
- **_Healthy Cooking Methods_**: Avoid frying or grilling red meat at high temperatures, which can create harmful compounds. Instead, opt for baking, steaming, or slow-cooking methods that preserve nutritional

content and reduce the production of carcinogenic substances.

Reducing red meat consumption and incorporating lean proteins like poultry, fish, tofu, and legumes can significantly benefit those managing uterine fibroids. Not only do these protein sources help maintain hormonal balance, but they also offer anti-inflammatory benefits that can support overall health. By making mindful dietary choices, you can take proactive steps toward managing fibroid symptoms and enhancing your well-being.

Increase Intake of Phytoestrogens

Phytoestrogens are naturally occurring plant compounds that can mimic the effects of estrogen in the body. They bind to estrogen receptors, potentially helping to balance hormone levels and reduce fibroid symptoms. Incorporating phytoestrogen-rich foods into your diet may support hormonal equilibrium and provide relief from fibroid-related discomfort.

Here's a detailed look at key sources of phytoestrogens:

Soy Products

Soy products are among the richest sources of phytoestrogens, specifically isoflavones, which are known for their ability to influence estrogen metabolism positively. Including soy in your diet can offer various health benefits:

- **Tofu**: This versatile soy product is made by coagulating soy milk and pressing the curds into soft white blocks. Tofu is not only rich in isoflavones but also provides high-quality protein, calcium, and iron. It can be used in a variety of dishes such as stir-fries, soups, salads, and even desserts.
- **Tempeh**: A fermented soybean product, tempeh is packed with isoflavones and probiotics, which support gut health. Its firm texture and nutty flavor make it an excellent meat substitute in sandwiches, burgers, and stews.
- **Soy Milk**: Made from soybeans, soy milk is a dairy-free alternative that contains isoflavones, protein, and essential vitamins like B12 and D. It can be used in smoothies, cereals, coffee, or as a substitute for cow's milk in baking and cooking.

Flaxseeds

Flaxseeds are another potent source of phytoestrogens, particularly lignans, which are known to have estrogenic and anti-estrogenic properties.

Adding flaxseeds to your diet can offer numerous health benefits:

- **Rich in Lignans**: Flaxseeds contain the highest concentration of lignans among plant foods. These

compounds can help balance estrogen levels by modulating estrogen activity in the body.
- **High in Omega-3 Fatty Acids**: Flaxseeds are an excellent source of alpha-linolenic acid (ALA), a type of omega-3 fatty acid that has anti-inflammatory effects, supporting overall health and reducing inflammation associated with fibroids.
- **Fiber-Rich**: The high fiber content in flaxseeds promotes digestive health and helps maintain stable blood sugar levels, contributing to hormonal balance.

How to Incorporate Flaxseeds into Your Diet:

- **Ground Flaxseeds**: To maximize absorption, consume ground flaxseeds rather than whole ones. Add them to smoothies, yogurt, and oatmeal, or sprinkle them over salads and roasted vegetables.
- **Flaxseed Meal**: Use flaxseed meal as a substitute for flour in baking recipes or as a thickening agent in soups and sauces.
- **Flaxseed Oil**: Incorporate flaxseed oil into salad dressings, dips, or drizzle it over cooked vegetables. Avoid using it for cooking at high temperatures, as it can degrade the beneficial compounds.

Other Sources of Phytoestrogens

While soy products and flaxseeds are among the most well-known sources, several other foods are rich in phytoestrogens and can be included in your diet for added benefits:

- *Legumes*: Chickpeas, lentils, and beans contain various types of phytoestrogens and provide protein, fiber, and essential nutrients.
- *Nuts and Seeds*: In addition to flaxseeds, sesame seeds, sunflower seeds, almonds, and walnuts are good sources of phytoestrogens.
- *Whole Grains*: Grains such as oats, barley, and rye contain lignans and other phytoestrogenic compounds.
- *Fruits and Vegetables*: Certain fruits (like apples, pomegranates, and berries) and vegetables (like carrots, yams, and sprouts) have phytoestrogenic properties.

Practical Tips for Increasing Phytoestrogen Intake

- *Diversify Your Sources*: Aim to include a variety of phytoestrogen-rich foods in your daily diet to benefit from their different compounds and nutrients.
- *Balance and Moderation*: While phytoestrogens can be beneficial, it's important to consume them in moderation as part of a balanced diet. Overconsumption can have varying effects, so it's best to consult with a healthcare provider for personalized advice.
- *Creative Cooking*: Explore new recipes and cooking methods to incorporate these foods into your meals.

Experiment with tofu stir-fries, tempeh sandwiches, flaxseed smoothies, and legume-based dishes.

Increasing your intake of phytoestrogens by incorporating soy products and flaxseeds into your diet can help balance hormone levels and alleviate fibroid symptoms. By diversifying your sources and consuming these foods in moderation, you can support overall hormonal health and enhance your well-being. Always consult with your healthcare provider to tailor dietary changes to your specific needs and conditions.

Foods to Eat for Managing Uterine Fibroids in Women

1. **High-Fiber Fruits and Vegetables**

    Incorporate a variety of high-fiber fruits and vegetables to help maintain hormonal balance and reduce inflammation.

    Examples:

    - *Leafy Greens*: Spinach, kale, Swiss chard, and collard greens
    - *Berries*: Strawberries, blueberries, raspberries, and blackberries
    - *Cruciferous Vegetables*: Broccoli, cauliflower, cabbage, and Brussels sprouts

- ***Citrus Fruits***: Oranges, grapefruits, lemons, and limes

2. **Whole Grains**

Whole grains are rich in fiber and essential nutrients, which can help regulate blood sugar levels and support overall health.

Examples:

- Brown rice
- Quinoa
- Barley
- Oats
- Whole wheat bread and pasta
- Healthy Fats

Consuming healthy fats, especially those from plant-based sources and fish, can help reduce inflammation and maintain hormonal balance.

Examples:

- ***Olive Oil***: Use extra virgin olive oil for cooking and dressings
- ***Nuts and Seeds***: Almonds, walnuts, chia seeds, and flaxseeds
- ***Fatty Fish***: Salmon, mackerel, sardines, and trout
- ***Avocados***

3. **Lean Proteins**

   Lean proteins are important for tissue repair and overall health. Focus on plant-based proteins, but include lean meats in moderation.

   Examples:

   - *Legumes*: Beans, lentils, chickpeas, and peas
   - *Poultry*: Chicken and turkey
   - *Eggs*: A versatile source of protein

4. **Anti-Inflammatory Herbs and Spices**

   Certain herbs and spices have anti-inflammatory properties that might help manage fibroid symptoms.

   Examples:

   - Turmeric
   - Ginger
   - Garlic
   - Cinnamon

5. **Low-Dairy Options**

   Some evidence suggests that reducing dairy intake may help with fibroid management. Opt for low-dairy or non-dairy alternatives.

   Examples:

   - Almond milk

- Coconut milk
- Soy milk
- Yogurt made from plant-based milks

6. Green Tea

Green tea contains antioxidants known as catechins, which may help reduce the size and number of fibroids.

How to Include:

- Drink one to two cups of green tea daily

Incorporating these foods into your diet can help manage uterine fibroids and promote better overall health. Remember to consult with a healthcare provider or a nutritionist for personalized dietary advice.

Foods to Avoid for Managing Uterine Fibroids in Women

1. Red Meat

Red meats, particularly those that are processed or high in fat, can contribute to inflammation and hormonal imbalances, potentially worsening fibroid symptoms.

Examples:

- Beef

- Pork
- Lamb
- Processed meats like sausages, hot dogs, and bacon

2. **Processed Foods**

Processed foods often contain unhealthy fats, sugars, and preservatives that can lead to inflammation and hormone disruption.

Examples:

- Packaged snacks (chips, cookies, crackers)
- Fast food
- Pre-packaged meals
- Sugary cereals

3. **High-Fat Dairy Products**

Full-fat dairy products can contain high levels of estrogen, which may exacerbate fibroid growth.

Examples:

- Whole milk
- Full-fat cheese
- Cream
- Butter

4. **Refined Carbohydrates and Sugars**

   Refined carbs and sugars can cause spikes in blood glucose levels, leading to increased insulin production and potential hormonal imbalances.

   Examples:

   - White bread
   - White rice
   - Pastries and sweets
   - Sugary drinks (sodas, energy drinks)

5. **Caffeine**

   High caffeine intake might contribute to the development of fibroids due to its effect on hormone levels.

   Examples:

   - Coffee
   - Energy drinks
   - Excessive amounts of black tea

6. **Alcohol**

   Alcohol consumption can interfere with liver function, which is crucial for hormone regulation. Additionally, some studies suggest a correlation between alcohol and an increased risk of fibroids.

   Examples:

- Beer
- Wine
- Spirits and liquors

7. **High-Salt Foods**

   Excessive salt intake can lead to water retention and increased blood pressure, which may worsen fibroid symptoms.

   Examples:

   - Canned soups and vegetables
   - Salty snacks (potato chips, pretzels)
   - Processed meats
   - Restaurant and fast food items

Avoiding these foods can help manage uterine fibroids and improve your overall health. Always consult with a healthcare provider or nutritionist to tailor dietary changes to your specific needs.

Supplements

In addition to a balanced diet and natural remedies, certain supplements can play a significant role in managing uterine fibroids. Here's an overview of essential vitamins, minerals, and anti-inflammatory supplements that can be beneficial.

Essential Vitamins and Minerals

Vitamin D

- ***Benefits***: Vitamin D is crucial for maintaining hormonal balance and may help reduce the size and number of fibroids. It supports immune function and has anti-inflammatory properties.
- ***Sources***: While sunlight is a natural source of Vitamin D, supplementation might be necessary, especially in areas with limited sun exposure or during the winter months.
- ***Dosage***: The recommended daily allowance (RDA) for most adults is 600-800 IU, but some studies suggest higher doses (1,000-2,000 IU) might be more effective for fibroid management. Always consult a healthcare provider for personalized dosage.

Omega-3 Fatty Acids

- ***Benefits***: Omega-3 fatty acids have powerful anti-inflammatory effects, which can help manage fibroid symptoms. They also support overall cardiovascular health and hormone regulation.
- ***Sources***: Found in fatty fish (like salmon, mackerel, and sardines), flaxseeds, chia seeds, and walnuts. Fish oil supplements are a common way to ensure adequate intake.
- ***Dosage***: A typical dose is 1,000 mg of combined EPA and DHA (the active components of omega-3s) per

day. Higher doses might be recommended based on individual needs.

Anti-Inflammatory Supplements

Turmeric

- ***Benefits***: Turmeric contains curcumin, which has potent anti-inflammatory and antioxidant properties. It can help reduce inflammation associated with fibroids and support overall liver health.
- ***Forms***: Available as capsules, tablets, or powders. It can also be consumed as a spice in food or as turmeric tea.
- ***Dosage***: Standardized turmeric extract typically contains 95% curcuminoids. A typical dose ranges from 500-2,000 mg per day, divided into multiple doses. For better absorption, take it with black pepper or a fat source, as curcumin is fat-soluble.

Ginger

- ***Benefits***: Ginger is another effective anti-inflammatory agent that can help alleviate pain and reduce inflammation. It also aids in digestion and boosts immunity.
- ***Forms***: Available fresh, dried, ground, or as capsules and extracts. Ginger tea is a popular way to consume it.

- ***Dosage***: For supplements, a typical dose ranges from 1,000-2,000 mg per day. Fresh ginger can be consumed by adding a few slices to hot water or incorporating it into meals.

Integrating Supplements Safely
- ***Consultation***: Always consult with a healthcare provider before starting any new supplement regimen, especially if you are taking other medications or have underlying health conditions.
- ***Quality***: Choose high-quality supplements from reputable brands to ensure purity and potency.
- ***Monitoring***: Keep track of any changes in symptoms or side effects and report them to your healthcare provider.
- ***Consistency***: Supplements typically need to be taken consistently over time to see benefits. Follow the recommended dosage guidelines and maintain regular intake for the best results.

By incorporating these essential vitamins, minerals, and anti-inflammatory supplements into your daily routine, you can effectively support the management of uterine fibroids and promote overall health.

Sample Recipes of Anti-inflammatory Food Diet to Manage Uterine Fibroids

To help you integrate these anti-inflammatory foods into your diet, here are a few simple recipe ideas:

Berry and Spinach Smoothie

Ingredients:

- 1 cup spinach
- 1/2 cup mixed berries (strawberries, blueberries, raspberries)
- 1 banana
- 1 cup unsweetened almond milk
- 1 tbsp chia seeds

Instructions:

1. In a blender, combine spinach and berries.
2. Add in the banana, almond milk, and chia seeds.
3. Blend until smooth.
4. Enjoy as a refreshing and anti-inflammatory breakfast or snack!

Quinoa and Veggie Salad

Ingredients:

- 1 cup cooked quinoa
- 1/2 cup cherry tomatoes, halved
- 1 cucumber, diced
- 1/4 cup red onion, chopped
- 1 avocado, sliced
- 2 tbsp olive oil
- Juice of 1 lemon
- Salt and pepper to taste

Instructions:

1. In a large bowl, combine quinoa, cherry tomatoes, cucumber, red onion, and avocado.
2. Drizzle with olive oil and lemon juice.
3. Season with salt and pepper to taste.
4. Toss until well combined.
5. Serve as a side dish or add in some grilled chicken for a complete meal.

Turmeric and Ginger Roasted Carrots

Ingredients:

- 1 lb carrots, peeled and cut into sticks
- 1 tbsp olive oil
- 1 tsp turmeric powder
- 1 tsp ground ginger
- Salt and pepper to taste

Instructions:

1. Preheat oven to 400°F.
2. In a bowl, mix together olive oil, turmeric powder, ground ginger, salt, and pepper.
3. Add in the carrot sticks and toss until well coated.
4. Spread out in a single layer on a baking sheet.
5. Roast for 20 minutes or until carrots are tender.
6. Serve as a tasty and anti-inflammatory side dish!

Salmon with Lemon and Dill

Ingredients:

- 4 salmon fillets
- 2 tbsp fresh dill, chopped
- 1 lemon, sliced
- 2 garlic cloves, minced
- 2 tbsp olive oil
- Salt and pepper to taste

Instructions:

1. Preheat oven to 375°F.
2. In a small bowl, mix together chopped dill, minced garlic, olive oil, salt, and pepper.
3. Place salmon fillets on a baking dish lined with parchment paper.
4. Spread the dill mixture evenly over each fillet.
5. Top each fillet with lemon slices.
6. Bake for 15-20 minutes or until salmon is cooked through.
7. Serve with quinoa and veggie salad for a complete anti-inflammatory meal!

Sweet Potato and Black Bean Tacos

Ingredients:

- 2 large sweet potatoes, peeled and cubed
- 1 can black beans, drained and rinsed
- 1 tsp cumin
- 1 tsp paprika
- 1/2 tsp chili powder
- 8 small corn tortillas
- 1 avocado, sliced
- Fresh cilantro for garnish

Instructions:

1. In a pot of boiling water, cook sweet potato cubes until tender.
2. Drain and set aside.
3. In a pan, heat black beans with cumin, paprika, and chili powder until warm.
4. Mash the sweet potatoes and mix in with the black bean mixture.
5. Warm tortillas in a separate pan.
6. Assemble tacos with sweet potato and black bean mixture, avocado slices, and fresh cilantro on top.
7. Enjoy these delicious vegetarian tacos as an anti-inflammatory dinner option!

Kale and Chickpea Stir-Fry

Ingredients:

- 2 cups kale, chopped
- 1 can chickpeas, drained and rinsed
- 1 red bell pepper, sliced
- 1 onion, chopped
- 2 garlic cloves, minced
- 2 tbsp olive oil
- 1 tsp cumin
- Salt and pepper to taste

Instructions:

1. In a large pan, heat olive oil over medium-high heat.
2. Add in chopped onions and sauté for 2 minutes.
3. Add in minced garlic and cook for an additional minute.
4. Stir in red bell peppers and cook for 2-3 minutes until slightly softened.
5. Mix in chickpeas and cumin, cooking for another 2-3 minutes.
6. Finally, add in the chopped kale and stir-fry everything together for about 5 minutes or until the kale is wilted.
7. Season with salt and pepper to taste before serving as a nutritious anti-inflammatory meal!

Avocado and Tomato Salad

Ingredients:

- 2 avocados, diced
- 1 pint cherry tomatoes, halved
- 1/4 cup red onion, chopped
- 2 tbsp olive oil
- Juice of 1 lime
- Salt and pepper to taste

Instructions:

1. In a large bowl, mix together diced avocados, halved cherry tomatoes, and chopped red onion.
2. In a separate small bowl, whisk together olive oil and lime juice.
3. Pour dressing over the avocado and tomato mixture and gently toss to coat evenly.
4. Season with salt and pepper to taste before serving as a refreshing salad packed with anti-inflammatory nutrients!

Lentil and Vegetable Soup

Ingredients:

- 1 cup lentils, rinsed
- 1 onion, chopped
- 2 carrots, diced
- 2 celery stalks, diced
- 2 garlic cloves, minced
- 1 can diced tomatoes
- 4 cups vegetable broth
- 1 tsp turmeric powder
- 1 tsp cumin
- Salt and pepper to taste

Instructions:

1. In a large pot, sauté chopped onions, diced carrots, and celery in olive oil over medium heat for 5 minutes.
2. Add in minced garlic and cook for an additional minute.
3. Stir in rinsed lentils, canned diced tomatoes, vegetable broth, turmeric powder, and cumin.
4. Bring soup to a boil then reduce heat to low and let simmer for 20-25 minutes or until lentils are tender.
5. Season with salt and pepper to taste before serving as a hearty anti-inflammatory meal!

Blueberry Chia Seed Pudding

Ingredients:

- 1/2 cup chia seeds
- 2 cups unsweetened almond milk
- 1 tbsp honey or maple syrup
- 1 cup fresh blueberries

Instructions:

1. In a large bowl, mix together chia seeds, almond milk, and sweetener of choice.
2. Let the mixture sit for 10 minutes to allow the chia seeds to expand and thicken.
3. Stir in fresh blueberries before pouring the pudding into individual jars or bowls.
4. Refrigerate for at least 4 hours or overnight to set.
5. Serve as a delicious anti-inflammatory breakfast option loaded with antioxidants and omega-3 fatty acids!

Cucumber and Mint Infused Water

Ingredients:

- 1 cucumber, sliced
- 1 handful fresh mint leaves
- 1 liter water

Instructions:

1. In a large pitcher, add sliced cucumbers and mint leaves.
2. Pour water over the ingredients and stir to combine.
3. Let the mixture sit in the fridge for at least an hour or overnight to allow the flavors to infuse.
4. Serve as a refreshing anti-inflammatory drink that can help reduce inflammation and aid in digestion!

Grass-fed Beef Stew

Ingredients:

- 1 lb grass-fed beef, cubed
- 2 tbsp avocado oil
- 1 onion, chopped
- 3 cloves garlic, minced
- 4 carrots, peeled and chopped
- 4 potatoes, peeled and diced
- 2 cups beef broth
- 1 tsp dried thyme
- Salt and pepper to taste

Instructions:

1. Heat avocado oil in a large pot over medium heat.
2. Add in cubed beef and cook until browned on all sides.
3. Stir in chopped onions and minced garlic, cooking for an additional minute.
4. Add in carrots and potatoes, followed by beef broth and dried thyme.
5. Bring to a boil, then reduce heat and let simmer for 1 hour or until beef is tender.
6. Season with salt and pepper to taste.
7. Serve as a hearty and anti-inflammatory meal that is packed with protein, vitamins, and minerals!

Grilled Chicken Salad

Ingredients:

- 4 boneless, skinless chicken breasts
- Salt and pepper to taste
- 1 tbsp olive oil
- 8 cups mixed greens
- 1 cup cherry tomatoes, halved
- 1 avocado, diced
- 1/2 red onion, thinly sliced

Instructions:

1. Preheat the grill to medium heat.
2. Season chicken breasts with salt and pepper on both sides.
3. Drizzle olive oil over the chicken breasts and rub to evenly coat.
4. Place chicken on grill and cook for 6-8 minutes on each side or until fully cooked.
5. Let chicken cool before slicing into strips.
6. In a large bowl, mix together mixed greens, cherry tomatoes, avocado, and red onion.
7. Top with sliced grilled chicken.
8. Serve as a delicious anti-inflammatory meal packed with protein, healthy fats, and antioxidants!

Buckwheat Pancakes

Ingredients:

- 1 cup buckwheat flour
- 1 tsp baking powder
- 1/4 tsp salt
- 2 tbsp maple syrup, plus more for serving
- 1 egg, beaten
- 1 cup milk (dairy or non-dairy)
- 1/2 cup fresh blueberries

Instructions:

1. In a large mixing bowl, combine buckwheat flour, baking powder, and salt.
2. In a separate bowl, whisk together maple syrup and egg.
3. Gradually add in the milk while whisking until well combined.
4. Slowly pour the wet mixture into the dry mixture and stir until just combined. Do not overmix.
5. Heat a large skillet or griddle over medium heat and lightly grease with cooking spray or butter.
6. Pour 1/4 cup of batter onto the skillet for each pancake.
7. Place a few blueberries on top of each pancake.
8. Cook until bubbles form on the surface, then flip and cook for an additional minute on the other side.

9. Serve hot with a drizzle of maple syrup for a delicious anti-inflammatory breakfast option that is also gluten-free and packed with antioxidants from the blueberries!
10. Optional: Add some ground flaxseed to the batter for an extra boost of anti-inflammatory omega-3 fatty acids.

Baked Salmon with Quinoa

Ingredients:

- 4 salmon fillets
- Salt and pepper to taste
- 1 tbsp olive oil
- 1 cup quinoa, cooked
- 1 cup cherry tomatoes, halved
- 1/2 red onion, diced
- 1/4 cup chopped fresh parsley

Instructions:

1. Preheat oven to 375°F.
2. Season salmon fillets with salt and pepper on both sides.
3. Drizzle olive oil over the fillets and rub to evenly coat.
4. Place salmon on a baking sheet lined with parchment paper.
5. Bake for 12-15 minutes or until fully cooked.
6. In a large bowl, mix together cooked quinoa, cherry tomatoes, red onion, and parsley.
7. Serve salmon on top of the quinoa mixture for a balanced and anti-inflammatory meal.
8. Enjoy the heart-healthy omega-3 fatty acids in salmon along with the anti-inflammatory properties of quinoa and vegetables!

Tofu Stir-Fry

Ingredients:

- 1 package extra-firm tofu, drained and pressed
- Salt and pepper to taste
- 1 tbsp olive oil
- 2 cloves garlic, minced
- 1 inch ginger, grated
- 1 cup broccoli florets
- 1 red bell pepper, sliced
- 1 carrot, sliced into thin rounds
- 1/4 cup low sodium soy sauce or tamari

Instructions:

1. Cut the pressed tofu into cubes.
2. Season with salt and pepper.
3. In a large pan over medium heat, add olive oil and sauté garlic and ginger for about a minute.
4. Add in the tofu and cook until lightly browned on all sides.
5. Remove tofu from the pan and set aside.
6. In the same pan, add broccoli florets, red bell pepper, and carrots. Sauté for 2-3 minutes until slightly tender.
7. Add the tofu back into the pan with the vegetables and pour in soy sauce or tamari. Stir to evenly coat everything in sauce.

8. Cook for an additional 2-3 minutes until heated through and the vegetables are fully cooked but still have a slight crunch.
9. Serve over rice or noodles for a satisfying anti-inflammatory meal filled with plant-based protein!

Lentil Soup

Ingredients:

- 1 cup dried lentils, rinsed and drained
- 1 tbsp olive oil
- 1 onion, chopped
- 2 cloves garlic, minced
- 2 carrots, peeled and chopped
- 2 celery stalks, chopped
- 4 cups low sodium vegetable broth or water
- Salt and pepper to taste

Instructions:

1. In a large pot over medium heat, add olive oil and sauté onions until translucent.
2. Add in garlic and cook for another minute.
3. Add in carrots and celery and cook for about 5 minutes until slightly softened.
4. Pour in the broth or water and bring to a boil.
5. Reduce heat to low and add in the lentils.
6. Let simmer for 20-25 minutes until the lentils are fully cooked and the soup has thickened.
7. Season with salt and pepper to taste.
8. Serve hot with crusty bread for a comforting and nutritious meal!

Berry and Spinach Smoothie

Ingredients:

- 1 cup fresh spinach leaves
- 1/2 cup mixed berries (blueberries, strawberries, raspberries)
- 1 banana
- 1 cup unsweetened almond milk
- 1 tbsp chia seeds

Instructions:

1. In a blender, add in spinach, mixed berries, banana, and almond milk.
2. Blend until smooth.
3. Add in chia seeds and blend for another 10-15 seconds.
4. Pour into a glass and enjoy a refreshing breakfast or snack packed with antioxidants and nutrients!

Quinoa and Kale Salad

Ingredients:

- 1 cup cooked quinoa
- 2 cups fresh kale, chopped
- 1/2 cup cherry tomatoes, halved
- 1/4 cup red onion, finely chopped
- 1 avocado, diced
- 2 tbsp olive oil
- Juice of 1 lemon
- Salt and pepper to taste

Instructions:

1. In a large bowl, combine cooked quinoa, chopped kale, cherry tomatoes and red onion.
2. Drizzle with olive oil and lemon juice.
3. Season with salt and pepper to taste.
4. Toss gently until well combined.
5. Top with diced avocado before serving.

Baked Salmon with Asparagus

Ingredients:

- 4 salmon fillets
- 1 bunch asparagus, trimmed
- 2 tbsp olive oil
- 2 garlic cloves, minced
- Juice of 1 lemon
- 2 tbsp fresh dill, chopped
- Salt and pepper to taste

Instructions:

1. Preheat oven to 375°F (190°C).
2. In a small bowl, mix together olive oil, minced garlic, lemon juice, and fresh dill.
3. Season salmon fillets with salt and pepper.
4. Place asparagus on a baking sheet and drizzle with half of the olive oil mixture.
5. Place salmon fillets on top of the asparagus and pour the remaining olive oil mixture over them.
6. Bake for 15-20 minutes until the salmon is fully cooked.
7. Serve hot.

Sweet Potato and Black Bean Stew

Ingredients:

- 2 large sweet potatoes, peeled and cubed
- 1 can black beans, drained and rinsed
- 1 red bell pepper, diced
- 1 onion, chopped
- 2 garlic cloves, minced
- 2 tbsp olive oil
- 1 tsp cumin
- 1/2 tsp smoked paprika
- 4 cups vegetable broth
- Salt and pepper to taste

Instructions:

1. Heat olive oil in a large pot over medium heat.
2. Add onion, garlic, and red bell pepper; sauté until soft.
3. Add sweet potatoes, cumin, and smoked paprika.
4. Pour in vegetable broth and bring to a boil.
5. Reduce heat and simmer for 20-25 minutes, until sweet potatoes are tender.
6. Stir in black beans and cook for an additional 5 minutes.
7. Season with salt and pepper before serving.

Turmeric and Ginger Lentil Soup

Ingredients:

- 1 cup red lentils, rinsed
- 1 onion, chopped
- 2 carrots, diced
- 2 celery stalks, diced
- 2 garlic cloves, minced
- 1 inch fresh ginger, grated
- 1 tsp turmeric powder
- 4 cups vegetable broth
- 1 can diced tomatoes
- 2 tbsp olive oil
- Salt and pepper to taste

Instructions:

1. Heat olive oil in a large pot over medium heat.
2. Add onion, garlic, ginger, carrots, and celery; sauté until soft.
3. Stir in turmeric and red lentils.
4. Add vegetable broth and diced tomatoes; bring to a boil.
5. Reduce heat and simmer for 25-30 minutes, until lentils are tender.
6. Season with salt and pepper before serving.

These recipes are designed to include anti-inflammatory and nutrient-rich ingredients that can help manage uterine fibroids and promote overall health.

7-Day Anti-Inflammatory Food Diet Sample Meal Plan

We have put together a 7-day sample meal plan to provide some inspiration for incorporating anti-inflammatory foods into your diet that will help you manage/prevent uterine fibroids. This plan includes a variety of plant-based meals that are easy to prepare and full of flavor.

Day 1

- *Breakfast*: Oatmeal with fresh berries and a handful of walnuts
- *Lunch*: Quinoa salad with mixed greens, chickpeas, cherry tomatoes, cucumber, and olive oil dressing
- *Snack*: Apple slices with almond butter
- *Dinner*: Grilled salmon, steamed broccoli, and brown rice

Day 2

- *Breakfast*: Smoothie with spinach, banana, almond milk, flaxseeds, and chia seeds
- *Lunch*: Lentil soup with a side of whole-grain bread

- **Snack**: Carrot sticks with hummus
- **Dinner**: Baked chicken breast, sweet potato, and sautéed kale

Day 3

- **Breakfast**: Greek yogurt with honey and mixed nuts
- **Lunch**: Turkey and avocado wrap with whole wheat tortilla
- **Snack**: Mixed fruit bowl (pineapple, grapes, and oranges)
- **Dinner**: Stir-fried tofu with mixed vegetables and quinoa

Day 4

- **Breakfast**: Whole grain toast with avocado and poached eggs
- **Lunch**: Spinach and mushroom frittata with a side salad
- **Snack**: Pear with a handful of almonds
- **Dinner**: Baked cod, roasted Brussels sprouts, and wild rice

Day 5

- **Breakfast**: Buckwheat pancakes with blueberries and a drizzle of maple syrup
- **Lunch**: Chickpea and vegetable curry with basmati rice

- **Snack**: Celery sticks with cottage cheese
- **Dinner**: Grass-fed beef stew with carrots and potatoes

Day 6

- **Breakfast**: Smoothie bowl with acai, granola, and fresh strawberries
- **Lunch**: Mixed bean salad with a lemon-tahini dressing
- **Snack**: Sliced cucumber with guacamole
- **Dinner**: Roasted turkey breast, green beans, and quinoa pilaf

Day 7

- **Breakfast**: Chia pudding made with coconut milk, topped with mango chunks
- **Lunch**: Grilled vegetable sandwich with whole grain bread
- **Snack**: Trail mix with dried fruit and pumpkin seeds
- **Dinner**: Shrimp stir-fry with broccoli, snap peas, and brown rice

Conclusion

Congratulations on making it to this part. Your commitment to understanding and managing your condition is a vital step toward taking control of your health. This guide has provided you with comprehensive insights into uterine fibroids, covering everything from their symptoms and causes to the various treatment options available.

Throughout this guide, you've gained knowledge about the nature of uterine fibroids, how to manage their symptoms, and the different treatments that can help you live a healthier, more comfortable life. Recognizing the symptoms—such as excessive menstrual bleeding, pelvic pain, and frequent urination—can help you catch fibroids early, leading to better outcomes.

Making simple changes to your diet and exercise routine can significantly impact your overall well-being. A balanced diet rich in fruits, vegetables, and whole grains, combined with regular physical activity, can support your body in managing fibroid symptoms. Non-surgical treatments like medications and procedures such as uterine artery embolization (UAE) offer effective options to control symptoms and shrink fibroids. Understanding these options allows you to make informed decisions about your care.

In some cases, surgery might be necessary. Myomectomy and hysterectomy are primary surgical treatments for fibroids, each with its benefits and considerations, especially regarding fertility and long-term health. The emotional aspect of dealing with fibroids should not be overlooked. Seeking support from friends, family, or a counselor can provide comfort and make navigating this journey easier.

Taking charge of your health is empowering. Staying informed about the latest research and treatment options ensures you are aware of the best choices for your situation. Regular visits with your healthcare provider will keep you updated. Developing a treatment plan tailored to your needs in collaboration with your healthcare team is crucial, as each woman's experience with fibroids is unique.

Tracking your symptoms through a diary can be invaluable for monitoring your condition. Documenting changes helps your doctor adjust treatments and find what works best for you. Complementary therapies like acupuncture, yoga, and mindfulness meditation can also play a role in reducing stress and improving overall well-being.

Facing uterine fibroids can feel isolating, but you're not alone. Building a strong support network makes a world of difference. Connecting with others who understand what you're going through provides emotional support and practical advice. Look for support groups focused on women's health or specifically on fibroids, whether online or local.

Raising awareness about uterine fibroids among your friends and family helps reduce stigma and encourages early diagnosis and treatment. Supporting organizations that fund fibroid research contributes to advocacy and donations, leading to better treatment options and improved care for all women affected by fibroids.

The future of fibroid management is promising. Ongoing research continues to uncover new treatments and better understand the causes of fibroids. By staying proactive, you can benefit from these advancements. Keeping an eye on clinical trials and new medical procedures unveils innovations that make treatment more effective and less disruptive.

A holistic approach to managing fibroids involves seeking healthcare providers who collaborate across specialties. Gynecologists, nutritionists, mental health professionals, and other specialists working together provide comprehensive care that addresses all aspects of your health.

Remember, you have the power to take control of your journey with uterine fibroids. Educating yourself, seeking support, and staying proactive transforms this challenge into an opportunity for empowerment and self-care.

Thank you for dedicating your time to reading this Uterine Fibroids Management Guide. We hope it has provided valuable insights and practical advice to help you manage your condition effectively. Your health and well-being are our top priority, and we wish you success and strength as you move forward.

If you have any questions or need further support, don't hesitate to reach out to healthcare professionals or support organizations dedicated to women's health and fibroids. You are not alone in this journey; a community is ready to support you every step of the way.

FAQs

What are uterine fibroids, and how common are they?

Uterine fibroids are non-cancerous growths that develop in or on the uterus. They vary in size and can cause a range of symptoms. Fibroids are quite common; up to 70-80% of women will develop them by age 50, though not all will experience symptoms.

What are the typical symptoms of uterine fibroids?

Common symptoms of uterine fibroids include excessive menstrual bleeding, extended durations, pelvic discomfort or pressure, frequent urination, difficulty emptying the bladder, constipation, and back or leg pain. Some women may not experience any symptoms at all.

How are uterine fibroids diagnosed?

Diagnosing uterine fibroids typically involves a pelvic exam followed by imaging tests such as an ultrasound or MRI. These tests help determine the size, number, and location of fibroids within the uterus.

What treatment options are available for managing uterine fibroids?

Treatment options for uterine fibroids range from lifestyle changes and medications to surgical procedures. Lifestyle changes include diet and exercise modifications. Medications can help control symptoms and shrink fibroids. Surgical options, such as myomectomy or hysterectomy, may be necessary in more severe cases. Non-surgical procedures like uterine artery embolization (UAE) are also available.

Can uterine fibroids affect fertility and pregnancy?

Yes, uterine fibroids can impact fertility and pregnancy. They may cause complications such as difficulty conceiving, miscarriages, or preterm labor. However, many women with fibroids can still conceive and have successful pregnancies. It's essential to discuss with your healthcare provider how fibroids might affect your specific situation.

Are there any natural or holistic approaches to managing fibroid symptoms?

Several natural and holistic approaches can help manage fibroid symptoms. These include maintaining a balanced diet rich in fruits, vegetables, and whole grains, regular exercise, stress-reducing practices like yoga and meditation, and complementary therapies such as acupuncture. Always consult your healthcare provider before starting any new treatment regimen.

When should I see a doctor about my fibroids?

If you encounter symptoms like excessive menstrual bleeding, intense pelvic discomfort, frequent urination, or difficulty emptying your bladder, it's important to visit a doctor. Furthermore, if you are trying to conceive and think fibroids may be impacting your fertility, seeking medical advice is vital. Identifying and treating fibroids early can enhance both their management and your overall quality of life.

References and Helpful Links

Uterine fibroids - Symptoms and causes - Mayo Clinic. (2023, September 15). Mayo Clinic. https://www.mayoclinic.org/diseases-conditions/uterine-fibroids/symptoms-causes/syc-20354288

Uterine fibroids - Diagnosis and treatment - Mayo Clinic. (2023, September 15). https://www.mayoclinic.org/diseases-conditions/uterine-fibroids/diagnosis-treatment/drc-20354294

American Fibroid Centers. (2024, February 6). Lifestyle Modifications and Self-Care for Uterine Fibroids | American Fibroid Centers. American Fibroid Centers. https://fibroidexpert.com/blog/lifestyle-modifications-self-care-for-uterine-fibroids/

Uterine fibroids: dos and don'ts. (2023, May 3). WebMD. https://www.webmd.com/women/uterine-fibroids/uterine-fibroids-dos-and-donts#:~:text=A%20recent%20study%20found%20that,could%20help%20improve%20your%20symptoms.

What are the risk factors for uterine fibroids? (2018, November 2). https://www.nichd.nih.gov/. https://www.nichd.nih.gov/health/topics/uterine/conditioninfo/people-affected

Iftikhar, N., MD. (2023, February 14). Shrinking Fibroids with Diet: Is It Possible? Healthline. https://www.healthline.com/health/fibroids-diet

Uterine fibroids | Office on Women's Health. (n.d.). https://www.womenshealth.gov/a-z-topics/uterine-fibroids#:~:text=Because%20no%20one%20knows%20for,anti%2Dhormone%20medication%20is%20used.

www.ingramcontent.com/pod-product-compliance
Lightning Source LLC
LaVergne TN
LVHW010404070526
838199LV00065B/5894